NOURISH

"A SIMPLE GUIDE TO A HEALTHIER, HAPPIER LIFE"

DR ROBERT MATTHEW

2 |ROBERT MATTHEW

TABLE OF CONTENT

INTRODUCTION

You might be wondering how is this book different from every other book I have read on diet and healthy lifestyle, you may even have been disappointed that none of what was suggested in the previous books worked and you might have come to a conclusion by asking yourself of what benefit is this book "NOURISH: THE SIMPLE GUIDE TO A HEALTHIER LIFESTYLE".

The book provides a very simple guide to living a healthy life, it also shares a lot of information on vitamins, nutrients, and supplements, and the natural sources to obtain the things

 The book is an introduction to how individuals can live healthier lives and the benefits of that it will also cover the importance of nourishment for overall health and well-being, the significance of food as medicine, and how it can affect our body, mind, and spirit.

It will also offer an overview of the book's topics, how it is structured, and what readers can expect to learn by reading it.

It will also briefly introduce the concept of mindful eating, whole foods, and the role of supplements in a healthy diet, as well as the link between food and mental health. And the emphasis of the book is to enable readers to make better choices in their diet and lifestyle to live a happier and more fulfilling life.

The book enlightens on the necessity of nourishment for overall health and well-being. It also discusses how the food we eat can affect every aspect of our lives, from physical health and energy levels to mood and mental clarity. The chapter could also highlight the increasing rates of chronic diseases such as obesity, type 2 diabetes, and heart disease, and how they are closely linked to poor dietary choices.

A section of the book covers the concept of food as medicine. This section provides examples of how different types of foods can support or impair various bodily functions. The chapter also covers the idea of nutrient density, which refers to the number of beneficial nutrients in a food compared to its calorie content.

There is a section of the book which is to empower readers to make healthier choices in their diet and lifestyle too to live a happier and more fulfilling life. It also provides an overview of the practical tips and strategies that will be discussed throughout the book, and how readers can apply them to their own lives.

The book also discusses how our modern lifestyle and food culture have led to an increase in processed foods and a decrease in nutrient-dense whole foods, which can have effects and lead to poor health consequences.

It also explains the idea that, while there is no one "perfect" diet that works for everyone, there are certain principles of healthy eating that can benefit everyone, such as emphasizing whole, unprocessed foods, eating a variety of different foods, and listening to your body's signals of hunger and fullness.

The book also touches on the importance of understanding the quality and source of the food we consume, including organic, non-GMO, and local options. It also explores the relationship between food, the environment, and sustainability.

Additionally, the book presents some statistics and research studies, to support the importance of eating nutrient-dense whole foods for health and well-being.

Finally, "NOURISH: THE SIMPLE GUIDE TO A HEALTHIER LIFESTYLE "summarizes the book's overall message and purpose, and explains how the information in the book will help readers achieve optimal health and happiness through nourishment by being fully present and engaged when eating, and being devoted to the texture and aromas of the food. Mindful eating can be an effective tool for breaking free from unhealthy eating patterns and learning to eat in a way that supports health and well-being.

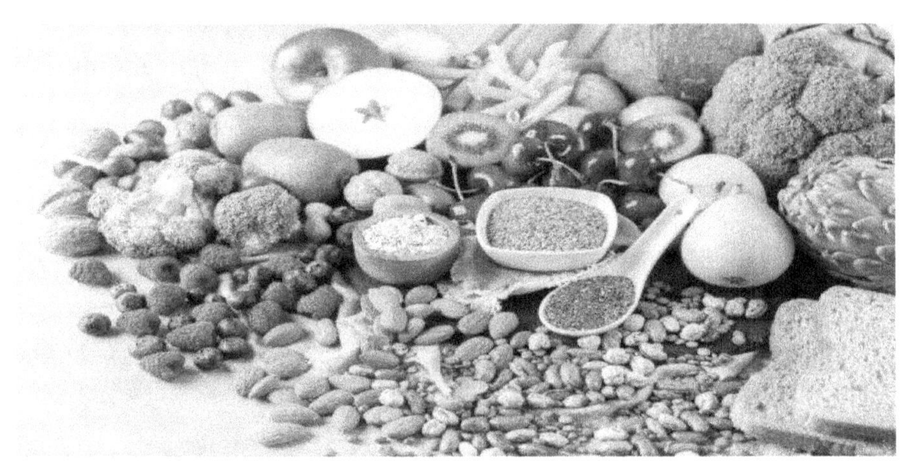

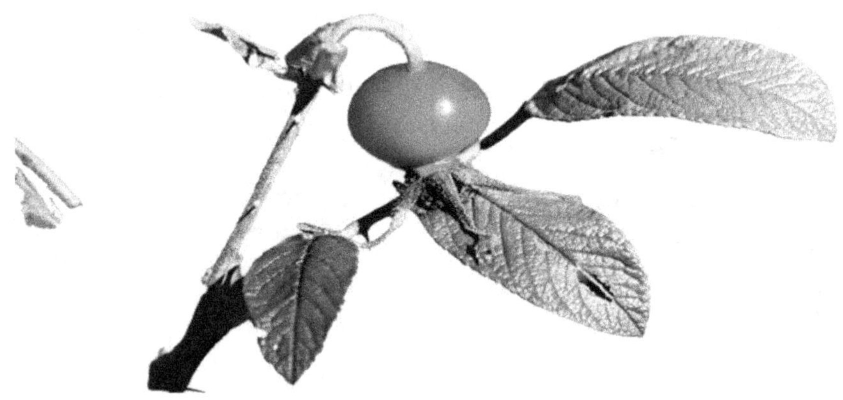

SOME EXAMPLES OF FRUITS FOR NUTRITION

10 |ROBERT MATTHEW

CHAPTER ONE

UNDERSTANDING THE BASICS OF NUTRITION

Nutrition is the science of how the body uses food to maintain health and prevent disease. It involves the intake of nutrients and other substances in food and their absorption, transport, metabolism, and excretion. The three main types of nutrients are carbohydrates, proteins, and fats, which provide energy and support the growth and repair of the body. Vitamins and minerals are also very important for proper bodily function.

In addition to the macronutrients (carbohydrates, proteins, and fats), there are also micronutrients, which include vitamins and minerals. These are required in smaller amounts but are still essential for maintaining good health.

A balanced diet includes a variety of nutrient-dense foods from all food groups, such as fruits, vegetables, whole grains, lean proteins, and healthy fats. It is also essential to reduce the consumption of added sugars, saturated fats, and sodium.

Proper nutrition is essential for maintaining good health and preventing chronic diseases such as obesity, heart disease, diabetes, and certain types of cancer. A healthy diet can also improve energy levels, mood, and cognitive function, as well as promote a healthy weight and overall physical well-being.

It is also important to pay attention to portion sizes and calorie intake, as overeating can lead to weight gain and other health problems. Consuming a balanced diet and engaging in regular physical activity can help maintain a healthy weight and prevent chronic diseases.

It's also important to note that certain individuals may have specific nutritional needs such as pregnant women, athletes, elderly people, and people with certain medical conditions. They may require different caloric intake, and nutrient intakes, and may need to consult a nutritionist or a doctor for a personalized plan.

The body needs a variety of vitamins and macro-nutrients to function properly. Here is a list of some of the most important vitamins and macro-nutrients, their sources, and their importance:

IMPORTANT VITAMINS AND MACRONUTRIENTS, SOURCES, AND IMPORTANCE

Carbohydrates: Carbohydrates are the body's main foundation of energy. They are discovered in foods like grains, fruits, vegetables, and legumes. Carbohydrates are important for maintaining blood sugar levels, fueling the brain and nervous system, and providing energy for physical activity.

Proteins: Proteins are essential for the growth, repair, and maintenance of the body's tissues. They are found in foods such as meats, fish, eggs, dairy, legumes, and some grains. Proteins are important for building

and repairing muscle, maintaining a healthy immune system, and producing enzymes and hormones.

Fats: Fats are a source of energy and also help absorb and transport fat-soluble vitamins. They are found in foods such as oils, butter, nuts, seeds, and avocados. Fats are important for providing insulation for the body's organs, maintaining healthy cell membranes, and supporting healthy hormonal functions.

Vitamin A: Vitamin A helps with vision, immune function, and cell growth. It's found in foods such as sweet potatoes, carrots, leafy greens, and dairy products.

Vitamin C: Vitamin C helps with the formation of collagen, which is important for skin, bones, and blood vessels. It also acts as an antioxidant, protecting the body from damage caused by harmful molecules. It's found in foods such as oranges, strawberries, bell peppers, and kale.

Vitamin D: Vitamin D helps the body absorb calcium and maintain healthy bones. It's found in foods such as fatty fish, egg yolks, and mushrooms. The body also produces vitamin D whenever the skin is visible to sunlight.

Vitamin E: Vitamin E acts as an antioxidant, protecting the body from damage caused by harmful molecules. It's found in foods such as almonds, sunflower seeds, and avocados.

Vitamin K: Vitamin K aids with blood coagulation and healthy bones. It's found in foods such as leafy greens, broccoli, and Brussels sprouts.

Calcium: Calcium is necessary for bone and healthy teeth. It's found in foods such as dairy products, leafy greens, and fortified foods.

Iron: Iron is vital for carrying oxygen into the bloodstream. It's found in foods such as red meat, leafy greens, and fortified cereals.

Magnesium: Magnesium helps with nerve and muscle function, blood sugar control, and bone health. It's found in foods such as leafy greens, nuts, and legumes.

Potassium: Potassium helps with nerve and muscle function and blood pressure control. It's found in foods such as bananas, potatoes, and leafy greens.

It's important to note that the body needs all these vitamins and macro-nutrients in the right balance and quantity, a deficiency or excess of any of these can lead to health issues. It's also recommended to consult a healthcare professional for more personalized advice and guidance on one's specific nutritional needs.

The chapter could also discuss micronutrients, which are the vitamins and minerals that the body needs in smaller amounts but are still essential for good health. It could provide an overview of the different types of micronutrients and their specific functions in the body, such as vitamin C for collagen production, and iron for oxygen transport.

The chapter could also cover the recommended daily allowances (RDAs) for different nutrients, and how they can vary depending on factors such as age, gender, and activity level. It could also discuss the idea of nutrient density and the importance of choosing nutrient-dense foods.

Additionally, the chapter could explain the concept of food groups, and how different types of foods can provide different types of nutrients. It could discuss how different types of fruits and vegetables provide different types of micronutrients, how lean meats and fish provide protein, and how legumes provide both protein and fiber.

Additionally, the chapter could provide an overview of some common nutrient deficiencies, and how they can affect the body. For example, anemia caused by iron deficiency, or osteoporosis caused by lack of calcium.

Finally, the chapter could encourage readers to consult with a registered dietitian or nutritionist for more personalized advice and guidance on their specific nutritional needs.

It could also be beneficial to provide some practical information such as how to read food labels, manage one's diet with dietary restrictions, and balance one's diet when eating out or ordering take-out.

WAYS IN WHICH MODERN CULTURE HAS LED TO AN INCREASE IN PROCESSED FOOD CONSUMPTION

Modern culture has led to an increase in processed food and a decrease in nutrient-dense whole foods in several ways:

Convenience: Processed foods are often more convenient to purchase, prepare, and consume than whole foods. They can be purchased in bulk, have a long shelf life, and often require little to no preparation.

Time-saving: With busy schedules and limited time, many people turn to processed foods as a quick and easy option for meals and snacks.

Advertising and Marketing: The food industry heavily markets and advertises processed foods, which can make them more appealing and desirable to consumers.

Affordability: Processed foods are often cheaper than whole foods, making them more accessible to people on a budget.

Availability: Processed foods are widely available in grocery stores, supermarkets, and fast-food chains, making it easy for people to purchase them regularly.

Palatability: Processed foods are often high in sugar, salt, and unhealthy fats, which can make them more appealing to taste buds, leading to overconsumption.

FACTORS THAT LED TO THE INCREASE IN PROCESSED FOOD CONSUMPTION

All these factors have led to an increase in processed food consumption while reducing the consumption of nutrient-dense whole foods, which are rich in vitamins, minerals, and other important nutrients. And as a result, it's leading to various health issues such as obesity, diabetes, heart disease, and nutrient deficiencies.

Changes in food production and distribution: With the rise of industrial agriculture and food processing, it has become easier and more profitable for food companies to produce and distribute processed foods on a large scale. This has led to a proliferation of processed foods in grocery stores and supermarkets.

Busy lifestyles: Modern culture places a high value on productivity and efficiency, which can leave people with little time for meal planning, cooking, and food preparation. Processed foods, which are often pre-packaged and require minimal preparation, have become an attractive option for many people.

Lack of food education: Many people are not taught how to cook or understand basic nutrition, leading to a reliance on processed foods. This can lead to poor food choices, overconsumption of certain macronutrients, and nutrient deficiencies.

Social norms: Eating processed foods has become a normalized part of modern culture and can be seen as a way to socialize, celebrate or reward oneself. These social norms can make it difficult for people to break away from processed foods and adopt a more nutrient-dense diet.

Food deserts: In some areas, particularly in low-income communities, access to whole foods can be limited, due to the lack of supermarkets or grocery stores in the area, so people living in these areas may have to rely on processed foods from nearby convenience stores.

All these factors combined have contributed to a situation where processed foods have become a staple of the modern diet, while nutrient-dense whole foods have become less prevalent.

This can lead to several health problems, including obesity, type 2 diabetes, heart disease, and nutrient deficiencies. Therefore, it's crucial to be more mindful of the foods we consume, and strive to include more nutrient-dense whole foods in our diet.

SOURCES OF NUTRIENTS AND VITAMINS NEEDED BY THE BODY AND TYPES

Many of the vitamins and macro-nutrients that the body needs can be sourced from a variety of foods. Here is a list of some of the main food sources for each nutrient:

Carbohydrates: Grains (such as rice, wheat, and oats), fruits (such as apples, bananas, and berries), vegetables (such as potatoes, sweet potatoes, and squash), and legumes (such as beans, lentils, and chickpeas).

Proteins: Meats (such as chicken, beef, and pork), fish (such as salmon, tuna, and cod), eggs, dairy (such as milk, cheese, and yogurt), legumes (such as beans, lentils, and chickpeas), and some grains (such as quinoa, amaranth, and teff)

Fats: Oils (such as olive, avocado, and coconut oil), butter, nuts (such as almonds, cashews, and peanuts), seeds (such as pumpkin, sunflower, and chia seeds), and avocados.

Vitamin A: Sweet potatoes, carrots, leafy greens (such as spinach and kale), and dairy products (such as milk, cheese, and yogurt).

Vitamin C: Oranges, strawberries, bell peppers, and leafy greens (such as kale and broccoli).

Vitamin D: Fatty fish (such as salmon and tuna), egg yolks, and mushrooms. The body is also one of the sources of vitamin D when the skin is exposed to sunlight.

Vitamin E: Almonds, sunflower seeds, and avocados.

Vitamin K: Leafy greens (such as spinach, kale, and collard greens), broccoli, and Brussels sprouts.

Calcium: Dairy products (such as milk, cheese, and yogurt), leafy greens (such as spinach and kale), and fortified foods (such as fortified orange juice and some types of tofu).

Iron: Red meat, leafy greens (such as spinach and kale), and fortified cereals.

Magnesium: Leafy greens (such as spinach and kale), nuts (such as almonds and cashews), and legumes (such as beans and lentils).

Potassium: Bananas, potatoes, and leafy greens (such as spinach and kale).

OTHER SOURCES OF MACRONUTRIENTS AND VITAMINS

It's also worth noting that some foods may have multiple sources of macro-nutrients and vitamins, for example, avocados are a source of healthy fats, vitamin E, and potassium. However, the bioavailability of the nutrient may vary depending on the food source, cooking methods, and other factors. It's always a good idea to have a balanced diet that includes a variety of different nutrient-dense foods to ensure that you're getting all the nutrients you need.

The recommended daily allowances (RDAs) for different nutrients are guidelines that indicate the minimum amount of a nutrient that a person should consume daily to maintain good health. The RDAs can vary depending on factors such as age, gender, and activity level.

Carbohydrates: The Institute of Medicine recommends that adults consume between 130-230 grams of carbohydrates per day, depending on the individual's energy needs.

Proteins: The RDA for protein is 0.8 grams per kilogram of body weight per day for adults. For example, a person who weighs 68 kg should consume about 55 grams of protein daily.

Fats: The RDA for fats is 20-35% of daily caloric intake

Vitamin A: The RDA for vitamin A is 900-700 micrograms per day for adult men and women, respectively.

Vitamin C: The RDA for vitamin C is 90 milligrams per day for men in adulthood and 75 milligrams per day for women in adulthood.

Vitamin D: The RDA for vitamin D is 600-800 International Units (IU) per day for adults.

Vitamin E: The RDA for vitamin E is 15 milligrams per day for adult men and women.

Vitamin K: The RDA for vitamin K is 120 micrograms per day for adult men and 90 micrograms per day for adult women.

FACTORS THAT AFFECT RECOMMENDED DAILY ALLOWANCES

Factors such as age, gender, and environment can affect the recommended daily allowances (RDAs) for different nutrients. Here's a bit more information on how each of these factors can affect nutrient needs:

Age: As people age, their nutrient needs can change. For example, older adults may need more vitamin D and calcium to support bone health, while infants and children have different nutrient needs than adults.

Gender: Men and women have different nutrient needs, for example, women require more iron than men because of menstrual blood loss.

Environment: Different environments can also affect nutrient needs. For example, people living in cold climates may need more vitamin D to support bone health, as vitamin D is synthesized in the skin in response to sunlight exposure. Similarly, athletes or people with higher physical activity levels may require more energy and protein to support muscle growth and recovery.

Pregnancy and lactation: Pregnant and breastfeeding women have higher nutrient needs, for example, pregnant women require additional folic acid, iron, and calcium to support the growth of the fetus.

Medical conditions: Some medical conditions may also affect nutrient needs. For example, people with celiac disease or gluten intolerance may require more vitamin B12, iron, and calcium. Similarly, people with diabetes may need to pay more attention to their carbohydrate intake.

It's also important to note that the RDAs are based on average needs and are meant to serve as general guidelines. Individual nutrient needs can vary depending on a person's specific health status, lifestyle, and dietary habits, it's always a good idea to consult a healthcare professional for personalized advice and guidance on nutrient needs.

DIFFERENCE FOOD GROUPS AND THEIR TYPES OF NUTRIENTS

Fruits: Fruits are a good source of carbohydrates, vitamins, and minerals, particularly vitamin C and potassium. They are also a good source of nutritional fiber.

Vegetables: Vegetables are a good source of carbohydrates, vitamins, and minerals, particularly vitamin A, vitamin K, and potassium They are also a good source of nutritional fiber.

Grains: Grains such as rice, wheat, oats, and barley are good sources of carbohydrates, vitamins, and minerals, particularly vitamin B, iron, and zinc. They are also a very good source of dietary fiber.

Protein: Protein foods include meats, fish, eggs, dairy, legumes, and some grains. They are a good source of essential amino acids, vitamins, and minerals, particularly iron, zinc, vitamin B12, and Vitamin B6.

Dairy: Dairy products such as milk, cheese, and yogurt are good sources of protein, carbohydrates, vitamins, and minerals, particularly calcium, vitamin D, and Vitamin B12.

Fats and Oils: Fats and oils such as olive, avocado, and coconut oil are good sources of energy and essential fatty acids such as

Omega-3 and Omega-6. They also help the body absorb and transport fat-soluble vitamins like vitamins A, D, E, and K.

It's worth noting that different foods within each group can provide a unique set of nutrients, so it's necessary to include a variety of foods from each group to ensure you are getting wide kinds of essential nutrients. Also, some foods may have multiple types of nutrients, for example, salmon is a good source of protein, omega-3, and Vitamin D. Therefore, it's important to have a balanced diet that includes a variety of different nutrient-dense foods from different food groups to ensure that you're getting all the nutrients you need.

NUTRIENTS DEFICIENCIES WITH EXAMPLES AND EFFECT

Nutrient deficiencies ensue when the body does not get enough of a definite nutrient from food. Common nutrient deficiencies include:

Iron deficiency anemia: Iron is essential for the production of hemoglobin, a protein in red blood cells that carries oxygen throughout the body. Iron deficiency anemia occurs when the body does not have enough iron to produce enough hemoglobin, which can lead to fatigue, weakness, and shortness of breath.

Vitamin D deficiency: Vitamin D is important for the absorption of calcium and the maintenance of strong bones. A deficiency can lead to weak bones, osteoporosis, and an increased risk of fractures.

Vitamin B12 deficiency: Vitamin B12 is important for the production of red blood cells, the proper functioning of the nervous system, and the maintenance of healthy DNA. A deficiency can lead to anemia, nerve damage, and cognitive impairment.

Iodine deficiency: Iodine is essential for the production of thyroid hormones, which regulate metabolism. Iodine deficiency can cause thyromegaly and hypothyroidism.

Folate deficiency: Folate (Vitamin B9) is important for the production of red blood cells and the proper functioning of the nervous system. A deficiency can lead to anemia, cognitive, impairment, and birth defects if occurs during pregnancy.

Calcium deficiency: Calcium is needed for durable bones. A deficiency can cause weak bones and a bigger risk of fractures.

Zinc deficiency: Zinc is important for the immune system, wound healing, taste, and smell. A deficiency can lead to an increased risk of infections and slow wound healing.

These are just a few examples of common nutrient deficiencies, and there are many other nutrients that the body needs to function properly. Nutrient deficiencies can have a variety of negative effects on the body, depending on the specific nutrient and the severity of the deficiency. In some cases, deficiencies can cause serious health problems if left untreated. It's important to have a balanced diet that includes a variety of nutrient-dense foods to ensure that you're getting all the nutrients you need. Consult a healthcare professional if you suspect you have a deficiency.

SOME COMMON NUTRIENT DEFICIENCIES AND EFFECTS

Iron deficiency anemia: Iron is essential for the production of hemoglobin, a protein in red blood cells that carries oxygen throughout the body. Iron deficiency anemia occurs when the body does not have enough iron to produce enough hemoglobin. Side effects of iron deficiency anemia include fatigue, weakness, and tininess of breath. It can also cause pale skin, rapid heartbeat, headaches, and difficulty maintaining body temperature. Iron deficiency anemia is particularly common in women due to blood loss during menstruation, and in people with a diet that is lacking in iron-rich foods.

Vitamin D deficiency: Vitamin D is important for the absorption of calcium and the maintenance of strong bones. A deficiency can lead to weak bones, osteoporosis, and an increased risk of fractures. Symptoms of vitamin D deficiency include muscle weakness, bone pain, and an increased risk of falls. Vitamin D deficiency is particularly common in people who have limited exposure to sunlight and in older adults.

Vitamin B12 deficiency: Vitamin B12 is important for the production of red blood cells, the proper functioning of the nervous system, and the maintenance of healthy DNA. A deficiency can lead to anemia, nerve damage, and cognitive impairment. Symptoms of vitamin B12 deficiency include fatigue, weakness, constipation, and nerve damage. Vitamin B12 deficiency is particularly common in people who follow a vegetarian or vegan diet and older adults.

Iodine deficiency: Iodine is essential for the production of thyroid hormones, which regulate metabolism. Iodine deficiency can cause thyromegaly and hypothyroidism. Symptoms of iodine deficiency include fatigue, weight gain, cold intolerance, and an enlarged thyroid gland. Iodine deficiency is particularly common in areas with iodine-poor soil.

Folate deficiency: Folate (Vitamin B9) is important for the production of red blood cells and the proper functioning of the nervous system. A deficiency can lead to anemia

HERE ARE SOME PRACTICAL TIPS FOR READING AND UNDERSTANDING FOOD LABELS AND MANAGING YOUR DIET:

Check the serving size and servings per container: The nutrition information on the label is based on a specific serving size, make sure you understand how much you are eating and adjust the information accordingly. If you are planning to eat more than one serving, you should multiply the nutrition information accordingly.

Look at the calories and macronutrients: The label will list the number of calories and macronutrients (carbohydrates, protein, and fat) per serving. This can help track your calorie and macronutrient intake, and for making sure you are getting the right balance of nutrients to meet your Check specific dietary needs

the vitamins and minerals: The label will list the number of certain vitamins and minerals in each serving, such as vitamin C, calcium, and iron. This can help ensure that you are getting enough of certain nutrients.

Pay attention to the ingredient list: Ingredient lists are listed in descending order by weight. Be aware of added sugars, sodium, and saturated fats, as well as any artificial ingredients or preservatives.

Look for health claims: Some food labels may include health claims such as "low-fat" or "high in fiber." These claims can be helpful, but it's important to read the nutrition information and ingredient list to get a full understanding of what the food contains.

Consider your dietary restrictions or allergies: If you have any dietary restrictions or allergies, it's important to look out for ingredients that you need to avoid, such as gluten or nuts.

Serving size and servings per container: The serving size and servings per container are important to understand because they give you an idea of how much you're eating. The nutrition information provided on the label is based on the serving size, so if you eat more than the serving size, you'll need to adjust the information accordingly. In addition, it's important to compare the serving size to your actual consumption.

Calories and macronutrients: The label will list the number of calories per serving as well as the number of carbohydrates, proteins, and fat. This information can help track your calorie and macronutrient intake, and for making sure you are getting the right balance of nutrients to meet your specific dietary needs. For example, if you are trying to lose weight, you'll want to pay attention to the number of calories and the amount of fat. If you're trying to build muscle, you'll want to pay attention to the amount of protein.

Vitamins and minerals: The label will list the number of certain vitamins and minerals in each serving, such as vitamin C, calcium, and iron. This information can help ensure that you are getting enough of certain essential nutrients.

Ingredient list: Ingredient lists are listed in descending order by weight. This means that the first ingredient on the list is the one that makes up the largest proportion of the product. Be aware of added sugars, sodium, and saturated fats, as well as any artificial ingredients or preservatives.

Health claims: Some food labels may include health claims such as "low-fat" or "high in fiber." These claims can be helpful, but it's important to read the nutrition information and ingredient list to get a full understanding of what the food contains.

Dietary restrictions or allergies: If you have any dietary restrictions or allergies, it's important to look out for ingredients that you need to avoid, such as gluten or nuts. Ensure to verify the ingredient list carefully.

It's important to remember that food labels are a guide and not a substitute for professional dietary advice. If you have specific dietary needs or concerns, it's always a good idea to consult a healthcare professional or a registered dietitian for personalized advice and guidance

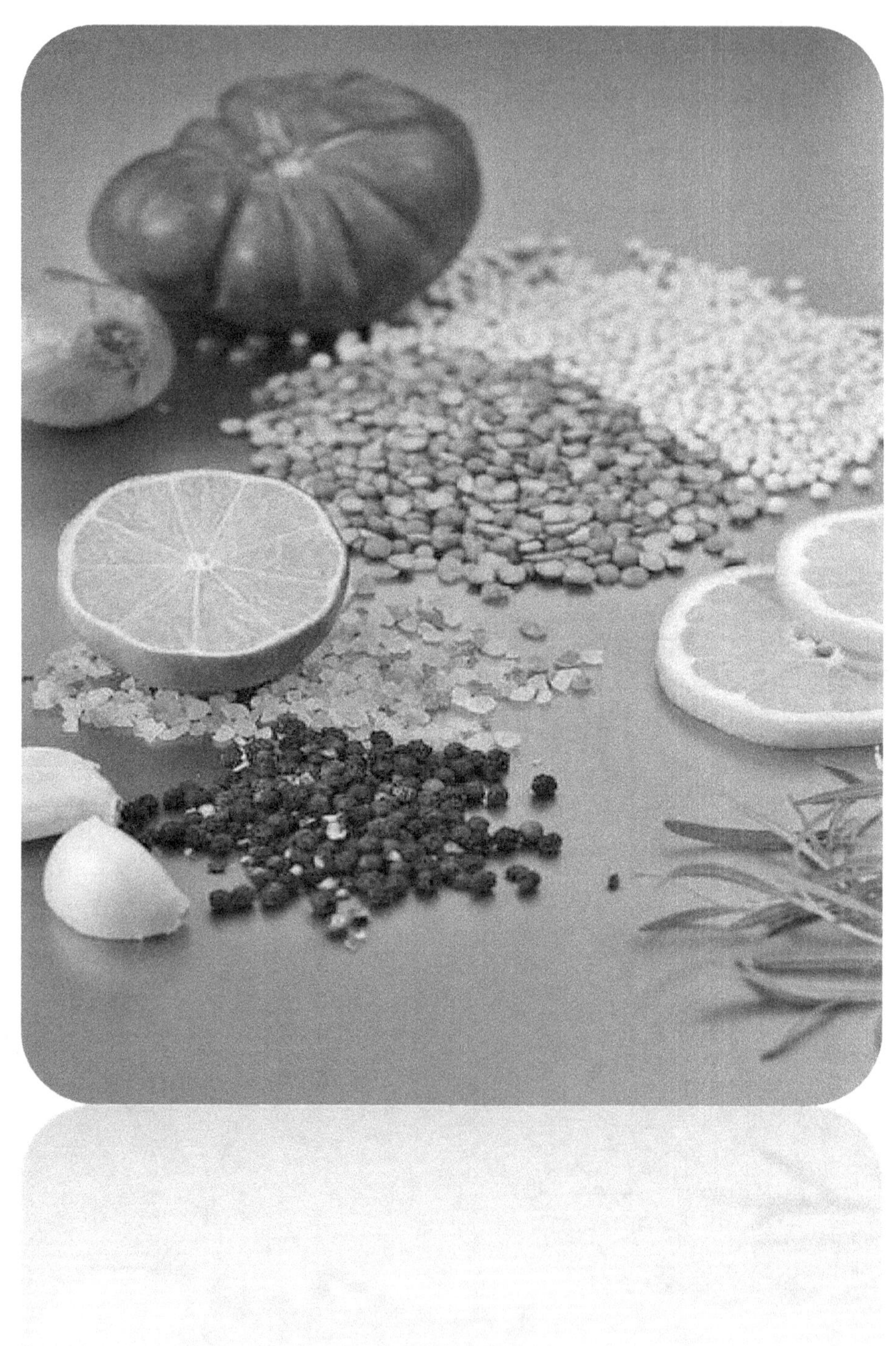

CHAPTER TWO

MINDFUL EATING IS KEY TO SUSTAINABLE WEIGHT LOSS

Weight loss refers to the process of losing body weight. This can be achieved by reducing the number of calories consumed, increasing the number of calories burned through physical activity, or a combination of both. When a person loses weight, they are losing a combination of body fat, muscle, and water.

WHAT IS WEIGHT LOSS

Weight loss occurs when the body is in a state of calorie deficit, which means that the body is burning more calories than it is taking in. The body will start to burn stored fat for energy, which results in the shrinkage of fat cells and weight loss. Additionally, when you increase physical activity, you burn more calories, which can also lead to weight loss.

To lose weight, it is essential to create a calorie deficit, which can be done by reducing calorie intake or increasing energy expenditure. A calorie deficit of 500-1000 calories per day is generally recommended for healthy weight loss, which can result in losing 1-2 pounds per week.

However, it's important to note that weight loss is not always linear and progress may not be always steady. Factors such as water retention, muscle gain, and hormone fluctuations can all affect weight loss progress. Additionally, weight loss should not be the only focus, it's important to think about overall health and wellness, not just the number on the scale. Therefore, it's important to seek guidance from a healthcare professional or registered dietitian to create a safe and sustainable plan for weight loss.

EATING HABIT

An eating habit refers to how a person eats, including the types of foods they choose to eat, the way they prepare and consume their food, and their attitudes and behaviors surrounding food. Eating habits can be influenced by a variety of factors, including cultural background, family traditions, personal preferences, and access to certain foods.

EXAMPLES OF EATING HABITS

Meal timing: This refers to when a person eats their meals and snacks. Some people may eat three large meals per day, while others may eat several small meals throughout the day.

Food choices: This refers to the types of foods a person eats, including whether they eat mostly plant-based foods or animal-based foods, and if they follow a particular diet such as a vegetarian or vegan diet.

Eating environment: This refers to the setting in which a person eats, including whether they eat at home, at a restaurant, or on the go, and if they eat alone or with others.

Eating behaviors: This refers to the attitudes and behaviors a person has towards food, such as if they eat when they are bored or stressed, if they eat quickly or slowly and if they pay attention to hunger and fullness cues.

Food preparation: This refers to how a person prepares their food, including if they cook at home or eat mostly processed foods.

CONCEPT OF EATING HABIT

Eating habits can vary widely among individuals and can change over time. Some eating habits may be healthy, while others may increase the risk of chronic health conditions such as obesity, heart disease, and diabetes. To maintain a healthy weight, it's important to adopt healthy eating habits which can be achieved by seeking guidance from a healthcare professional or registered dietitian.

Eating habits play a crucial role in sustainable weight loss. By making small, gradual changes to your eating habits, you can create a calorie deficit and lose weight healthily and sustainably. Here are a few ways that eating habits can lead to sustainable weight loss

WAYS EATING HABITS CAN LEAD TO WEIGHT LOSS

- Eating nutrient-dense foods: Focus on incorporating nutrient-dense foods into your diet, such as fruits, vegetables, lean proteins, and whole grains. These foods are typically lower in calories and high in essential nutrients, which can help keep you feeling full and satisfied while reducing your overall calorie intake.

- Portion control: Paying consideration to share sizes can aid you to control your calorie intake. By eating smaller portions, you can reduce the number of calories you consume without feeling deprived.

- Eating regular meals and snacks: Skipping meals can lead to overeating and make it harder to control your calorie intake. Eating regular, balanced meals and snacks throughout the day can help keep your hunger in check and prevent overeating.

- Mindful eating: Mindful eating means paying attention to your hunger and fullness levels, and eating in response to those cues. It also means savoring your food and being fully present while you eat. This can help you to better understand your body's signals and make more mindful choices about what and how much to eat.
- Avoiding processed foods and added sugars: Processed foods and foods high in added sugars are often high in calories and low in nutrients. Limiting these foods in your diet can help reduce your calorie intake and improve the overall quality of your diet.

By following these guidelines, you can make changes to your eating habits that will lead to sustainable weight loss. Additionally, it's important to seek guidance from a healthcare professional or registered dietitian to create a safe and sustainable plan for weight loss, as well as to monitor progress and make adjustments as necessary

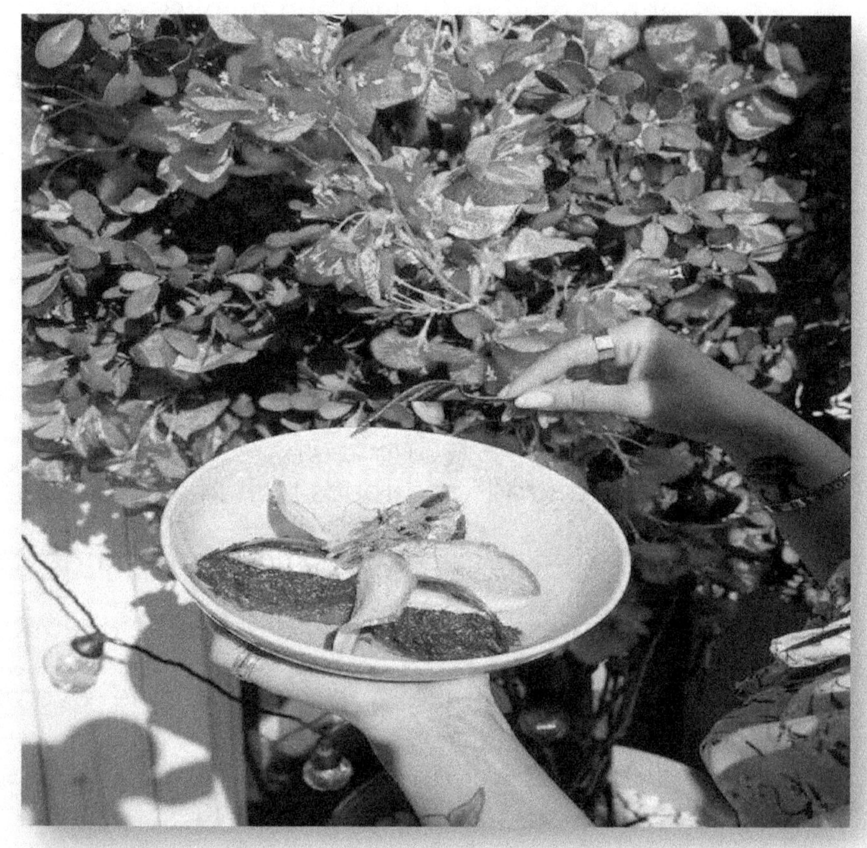

EXAMPLES OF HEALTHY UNPROCESSED FOOD

40 |ROBERT MATTHEW

CHAPTER THREE

IMPORTANCE OF WHOLE FOOD

Whole foods are foods that are minimally processed or unprocessed and retain most of their natural nutritional value. Whole foods are often considered to be healthier options than processed foods because they contain more vitamins, minerals, antioxidants, and other beneficial nutrients.

Eating whole foods, as opposed to processed foods, is important for maintaining a healthy diet. Whole foods are minimally processed and often contain more nutrients, vitamins, and minerals than processed foods. They also tend to be lesser in added sugars, sodium, and unwholesome fats. Consuming a diet rich in whole foods can help reduce the risk of chronic diseases such as heart disease, diabetes, and certain cancers. Additionally, whole foods can help with weight management and provide a feeling of satiety and energy. Overall, whole foods play a vital role in providing the essential nutrients that the body needs to function properly.

Another important benefit of whole foods is that they are often more satisfying and filling than processed foods. Whole foods often contain more fiber, which can help you feel full for longer periods. This can be beneficial for weight management and can help you avoid overeating. Additionally, whole foods tend to be less processed, meaning they are closer to their natural state, which can make them more nutrient-dense and flavorful. This can make it easier to enjoy healthy eating and maintain a healthy diet over the long term. Additionally, consuming whole foods can also help support a healthy gut microbiome, which is important for overall health and well-being.

EXAMPLES OF WHOLE FOOD

Fresh fruits and vegetables

Whole grains like brown rice, quinoa, and cereals

Legumes like beans, lentil plants, and pea plant

Nuts and seeds

Slim proteins like fish, chicken, and tofu

Dairy foodstuffs

IMPORTANCE OF WHOLE FOOD

Whole foods are often the building blocks of a healthy diet. They are high in fiber, vitamins and minerals, and other essential nutrients. Eating a diet rich in whole foods can help reduce the risk of chronic diseases, improve heart health, and support weight management. Whole foods are also often more satisfying than processed foods and can help to reduce cravings for sugar and other unhealthy foods.

It's important to note that some foods that are considered whole foods, like nuts, seeds, and avocado, are high in calories, so it's important to pay attention to portion sizes when incorporating them into your diet.

Whole foods are important for the body because they provide a wide range of essential nutrients that are needed for optimal health. Some of the specific benefits of consuming whole foods include:

BENEFIT OF CONSUMING WHOLE FOOD

Nutrient-dense: Whole foods are naturally nutrient-dense, meaning they are high in essential vitamins, minerals, and other beneficial compounds such as antioxidants and phytochemicals. These nutrients play important roles in maintaining good health, including supporting the immune system, promoting healthy digestion, and reducing the risk of chronic diseases.

High in Fiber: Whole foods are typically rich in dietary fibers which are important for maintaining a healthy gut, regular bowel movements, and lower cholesterol levels.

Promote Weight Management: Whole foods are often more satiating than processed foods, which can help with weight management. They are also typically lower in calories, making it easier to control calorie intake and create a calorie deficit for weight loss.

Support Heart Health: Whole foods, particularly fruits and vegetables, are rich in antioxidants and other beneficial compounds that have been shown to support heart health.

Eating a diet rich in whole foods can help lower blood pressure, reduce inflammation, and improve cholesterol levels.

Support Blood sugar control: Whole foods like whole grains, fruits, vegetables, and legumes are high in fiber, which can help slow down digestion and absorption of sugar, resulting in more stable blood sugar levels.

Encourage a varied diet: Eating a variety of whole foods can provide the body with a diverse range of nutrients and phytochemicals, which can promote overall health and well-being

By consuming a diet rich in whole foods, you can ensure that your body is getting the essential nutrients it needs for optimal health. Whole foods can also help you to feel more satisfied and less likely to crave unhealthy processed foods.

WHAT IS WHOLE FOOD

Whole foods are a good source of vitamins and minerals: Whole foods are rich in essential vitamins and minerals such as vitamin C, vitamin A, vitamin K, folate, potassium, and magnesium. These nutrients play a vital role in maintaining good health, including supporting the immune system, promoting healthy digestion, and reducing the risk of chronic diseases.

Whole foods are high in antioxidants: Whole foods such as fruits, vegetables, whole grains, and nuts are rich in antioxidants, which are beneficial compounds that protect the body from damage caused by free radicals. These antioxidants help to lower inflammation, prevent chronic disease, and reduce the risk of cancer.

Whole foods support digestion: Whole foods are typically high in fiber, which is important for maintaining a healthy gut, regular bowel movements, and reducing constipation. Whole foods also promote the growth of beneficial bacteria in the gut, which can help to improve digestion and boost the immune system.

Whole foods support mental health: Eating a diet rich in whole foods has been linked to improved mood, reduced stress, and better cognitive function. Whole foods are a good source of essential nutrients like omega-3 fatty acids and B vitamins, which are important for maintaining good mental health.

Whole foods are sustainable: Whole foods are often locally sourced, in season, and produced in a way that is less harmful to the environment. Eating whole foods can help to reduce the impact on the environment and promote sustainable living.

Whole foods are affordable: Whole foods are often less expensive than processed foods, especially when purchased in bulk or when in season. Eating whole foods can be a cost-effective way to maintain a healthy diet.

It's important to note that consuming whole foods alone doesn't guarantee optimal health, it's also important to pay attention to portion sizes and balance the diet with different types of nutrients, whole foods should also be combined with regular physical activity and a balanced lifestyle to achieve optimal health.

CHAPTER FOUR

THE ROLE OF SUPPLEMENTS IN A HALE AND HEARTY FOOD

Supplements can play a role in helping to fill any nutrient gaps in a person's diet. Whole foods are the best source of nutrients, however, it's not always possible to get all the nutrients that the body needs from diet alone. This is where supplements can be of immeasurable importance.

Some examples of when supplements may be necessary include:

Vegetarians and vegans may need to supplement with vitamin B12, as it is mainly found in animal products.

People who are lactose intolerant may need to supplement with calcium.

People who have difficulty taking in nutrients as a result of certain medical ailments may need supplements to meet their nutritional needs.

It's crucial to stress that supplements should not be a substitute for a healthy diet. They should be in place to supplement a healthy diet, not substitute for it.

It's also important to consult with a healthcare professional before starting any supplement regimen, as some supplements can interact with medications or have other risks.

A healthy diet provides the body with the necessary nutrients for optimal health and well-being. A healthy diet should include a balance of macronutrients (carbohydrates, proteins, and fats) and micronutrients (vitamins and minerals) and should be based on whole, unprocessed foods.

KEY COMPONENT OF A HEALTHY DIET

A variety of fruits and vegetables: Fruits and vegetables are rich in vitamins, minerals, and antioxidants, which are essential for maintaining good health. Aim to eat a variety of different colored fruits and vegetables to ensure that you're getting a wide range of nutrients.

Whole grains: Whole grains, such as brown rice, quinoa, and oats, are an important source of fiber and other essential nutrients. They are also less processed than refined grains, such as white flour and white rice, and can provide a slower release of energy.

Lean proteins: Lean proteins, such as fish, chicken, and tofu, are important for building and repairing tissues in the body. They also aid in making you feel filled and satisfied.

Healthy fats: Healthy fats, such as those found in avocados, nuts, and seeds, are important for maintaining healthy cholesterol levels and heart health.

Limited added sugars and sodium: Consuming large amounts of added sugars and sodium can contribute to chronic health conditions such as obesity, heart disease, and high blood pressure. It is important to limit the intake of these in a healthy diet.

Hydration: Drinking enough water is important for overall health and well-being.

It's important to note that a healthy diet is not a one-size-fits-all approach, different people have different nutrient needs based on their age, gender, activity level, and other factors. It's important to consult with a healthcare professional or registered dietitian to create a personalized and healthy diet plan.

WHAT ARE SUPPLEMENTS

A supplement is a product that is intended to supplement the diet and provide nutrients, such as vitamins, minerals, fibers, fatty acids, or amino acids, that may be missing or not consumed in adequate amounts in a person's diet. Supplements are available in many forms, such as tablets, capsules, soft gels, gel caps, liquids, and powders, and can be taken orally.

Some supplements are used to improve overall health and wellness, while others are used to target specific health conditions or deficiencies. It's important to note that supplements are not a substitute for a healthy diet and should not be used to replace the variety of foods that are important for a healthy diet. It is always best to consult a healthcare professional before taking any kind of supplement. Supplements can be classified into several categories based on their intended use, such as It's important to note that the effectiveness and safety of supplements can vary depending on the specific product, and some supplements may interact with medications or have side effects.

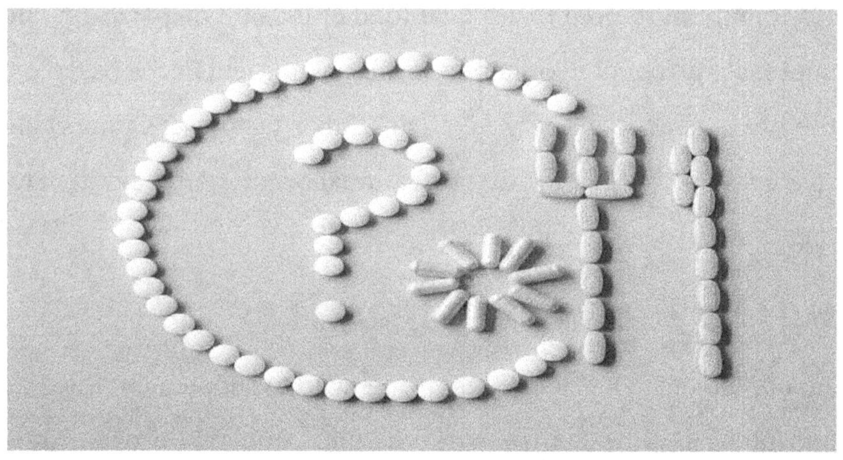

SOME SUPPLEMENT THAT AID NUTRITION

DIFFERENT TYPES OF SUPPLEMENTS

Multivitamins: These are supplements that comprise a combination of diverse vitamins and minerals. They are commonly used to help fill nutrient gaps in a person's diet.

Mineral supplements: These supplements contain individual minerals such as iron, zinc, or calcium. They are commonly used to correct mineral deficiencies in the diet.

Herbal supplements: These supplements contain plant-based ingredients, such as herbs, roots, or botanicals, and are used for their potential health benefits.

Protein supplements: These supplements are used to increase the intake of protein, which is important for building and repairing muscle tissue.

Probiotics: These supplements comprise live bacteria and yeast that are analogous to the useful microorganisms found in the human gut. They are commonly used to promote a healthy gut.

It's important to note that supplements are not intended to replace a healthy diet, and it's always best to try to get the nutrients you need from food, rather than supplements. It's also important to consult with a healthcare professional or registered dietitian before starting any supplement regimen, as they can interact with medications or have adverse effects on certain health conditions.

Supplements can play a role in a healthy diet by helping to fill nutrient gaps and ensure that the body is getting all of the essential vitamins and minerals it needs. However, it's vital to be aware that supplements should not be used as a replacement for healthy food. Eating a variety of nutrient-dense whole foods is the best way to meet your nutritional needs.

SITUATIONS WHERE SUPPLEMENT IS USEFUL IN A HEALTHY DIET

To correct nutrient deficiencies: Certain individuals may have a deficiency in specific nutrients, such as iron, vitamin D, or calcium. In such cases, a supplement may be necessary to correct the deficiency and promote optimal health.

To support specific health conditions: Certain supplements may be recommended to support specific health conditions, such as omega-3 fatty acids for heart health, or vitamin B12 for vegetarians and veggies who may be in danger of shortage.

To support athletic performance: Athletes may have increased nutritional needs, and some supplements like protein powder, or creatine, may be used to support muscle building and recovery.

To support weight loss: Some weight-loss supplements may contain ingredients that can help to suppress appetite or increase feelings of fullness, but it's important to note that there is no magic pill that will make you lose weight, and such supplements should be used with caution and under the guidance of a healthcare professional.

It's important to consult with a healthcare professional or registered dietitian before starting any supplement regimen, as they can interact with medications or have adverse effects on certain health conditions. They can also help you to determine if you have any nutrient deficiencies and if a supplement is necessary, and which type and how much of it you should take.

Supplements can be a valuable addition to a healthy diet, but it's important to remember that they are not a replacement for whole, nutrient-dense foods. The best way to meet your nutritional needs is by consuming a variety of nutrient-dense whole foods.

HERE ARE SOME FURTHER DETAILS ON THE ROLE OF SUPPLEMENTS IN A HEALTHY DIET:

They can help to fill nutrient gaps: A healthy diet should consist of a variety of nutrient-dense foods, but it can be difficult to meet all of your nutritional needs through diet alone. Supplements can help to fill nutrient gaps and ensure that the body is getting all of the essential vitamins and minerals it needs.

They can be used as a safety net: Even with a healthy diet, it's possible to fall short on certain nutrients, especially if you have a health condition or dietary restriction that affects nutrient absorption or utilization. In such cases, a supplement can provide an added safety net to ensure that the body is getting all the necessary nutrients.

They can be used for therapeutic purposes: Certain supplements may be used to address specific health concerns, such as omega-3 fatty acids for heart health, or probiotics for gut health. However, it's important to consult with a healthcare professional or registered dietitian to determine if a supplement is necessary and which type and how much of it you should take.

They can be used for convenience: Some supplements, such as protein powders, can be used as a convenient way to increase your protein intake, especially if you have a busy lifestyle or find it difficult to consume enough protein through diet alone.

It's important to note that not all supplements are created equal, and some may not be effective or may even be harmful. It's important to choose supplements from reputable sources, and also to check for any potential side effects or interactions with other medications or supplements you may be taking. It is also recommended to consult with a healthcare professional or registered dietitian to determine if a supplement is necessary and which type and how much of it you should take.

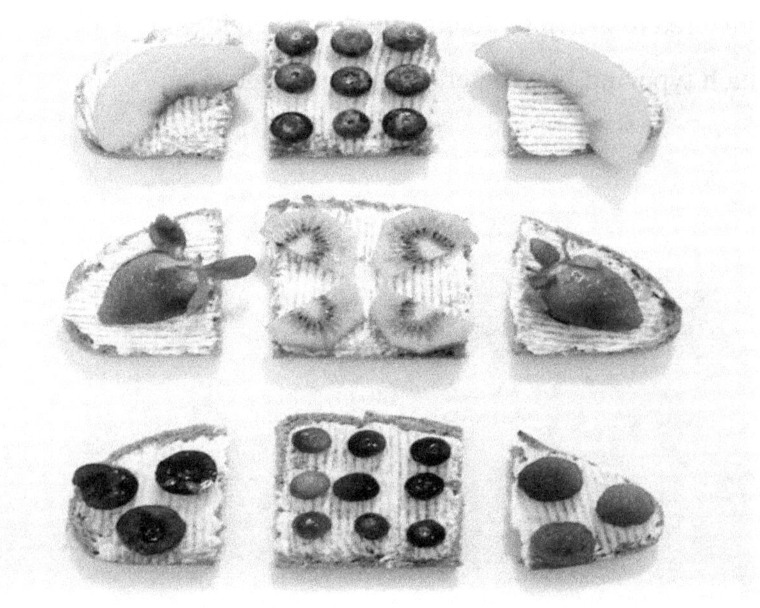

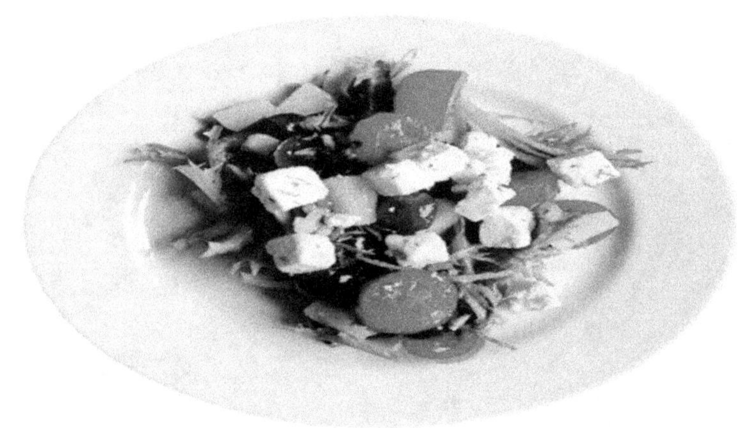

DIET

THAT PROMOTE GOOD HEALTH AND LIFESTYLE

56 |ROBERT MATTHEW

CHAPTER FIVE

NOURISHING YOUR BODY, A GUIDE TO PHYSICAL FITNESS

To nourish your body means to provide it with the necessary nutrients, vitamins, minerals, and other essential substances it needs to function properly and maintain optimal health. Nourishing your body includes providing it with the energy it needs through carbohydrates, fats, and proteins, as well as providing it with vitamins,

minerals, and other essential nutrients that are needed for the growth, repair, and maintenance of the body.

Nourishing your body also includes providing it with an adequate amount of fluids, such as water, to help regulate body temperature and support the body's metabolism. It also includes providing the body with adequate rest and sleep to support the body's recovery and repair processes.

To nourish your body, it's important to eat a balanced diet that includes a variety of whole, nutrient-dense foods. This means consuming foods that are high in vitamins, minerals, antioxidants, and other beneficial compounds, as well as foods that are low in added sugars, saturated fats, and sodium.

It's also important to pay attention to portion sizes and to practice mindful eating habits, such as eating slowly and savoring each bite, to ensure that you are eating the right amount of food for your body's needs. Additionally, regular physical activity and maintaining a healthy lifestyle are also important for nourishing the body.

In summary, nourishing your body means providing it with everything it needs for optimal health and well-being through a balanced diet, regular physical activity, hydration, sleep, and a healthy lifestyle.

WHAT IS PHYSICAL FITNESS

Physical fitness refers to the ability of the body to perform various physical tasks and activities with ease, efficiency, and without undue fatigue. It is a measure of the body's overall health and well-being and encompasses several

DIFFERENT COMPONENTS OF PHYSICAL FITNESS:

Cardiorespiratory fitness: This refers to the ability of the heart, lungs, and blood vessels to deliver oxygen and nutrients to the body's tissues during physical activity.

Muscular fitness: This refers to the strength, endurance, and tone of the muscles.

Flexibility: This refers to the capability of the joints to interchange through a full variety of motions.

Body composition: This refers to the proportion of lean body mass (muscles, bones, organs) to body fat.

Balance and coordination: This refers to the ability to maintain stability and control of the body during various movements.

Physical fitness can be improved through regular physical activity and exercise, as well as through a healthy diet and lifestyle. Regular exercises, such as strength training, cardio, and stretching, can help to improve cardiovascular fitness, muscular fitness, flexibility, and body composition, while also reducing the risk of chronic diseases, such as heart disease and obesity.

It's important to note that physical fitness isn't only about looking good, but it's a measure of your overall health and well-being.

Regular physical activity and exercise can help to improve overall health, boost mood, and reduce the risk of chronic diseases. It's important to consult with a healthcare professional or a personal trainer to design a safe and effective exercise program that meets your needs and goals.

RELATIONSHIP BETWEEN PHYSICAL FITNESS AND NOURISHMENT

The relationship between nourishment and physical fitness is closely linked, as both are essential for maintaining optimal health and well-being. Proper nourishment provides the body with the necessary nutrients, vitamins, and minerals to perform at its best, while physical fitness allows the body to put those nutrients to use through movement and activity.

Proper nourishment is essential for physical fitness because it provides the body with the energy it needs to perform physical activity. Carbohydrates, fats, and proteins are the main sources of energy for the body, and a diet that is deficient in these macronutrients can lead to fatigue and decreased physical performance. Adequate hydration is also important for physical fitness, as it helps to regulate body temperature and support the body's metabolism during exercise.

Physical fitness, on the other hand, also supports proper nourishment by helping to maintain healthy body weight and composition. Regular exercise can help to increase muscle mass, which in turn increases metabolism, leading to improved energy balance and weight management. Exercise also helps to reduce the risk of chronic diseases such as obesity, type 2 diabetes, and heart disease, which are all linked to poor nutrition and a sedentary lifestyle.

Additionally, the connection between nourishment and physical fitness also includes the mental and emotional aspects. A well-nourished body with enough energy and nutrients can help to improve mood, reduce stress and anxiety, and increase overall feelings of well-being. Physical fitness also has positive effects on mental health, by releasing endorphins that can improve mood and reduce stress.

In summary, proper nourishment and physical fitness are closely linked, as proper nourishment provides the body with the necessary nutrients to perform at its best, while physical fitness allows the body to put those nutrients to use through movement and activity. A well-nourished body with adequate physical activity results in optimal health and well-being, both physically and mentally.

Nourishment can be considered a guide to physical fitness because it provides the body with the necessary nutrients, vitamins, and minerals to support and maintain optimal physical performance. Proper nourishment is essential for physical fitness because it provides the body with the energy it needs to perform physical activity and repair and rebuild muscle tissue after exercise.

A balanced diet that includes a variety of whole, nutrient-dense foods can help to provide the body with the necessary energy, vitamins, minerals, and other essential nutrients it needs to support physical fitness. Adequate intake of macronutrients such as carbohydrates, fats, and proteins, is necessary for energy production, while micronutrients such as vitamins and minerals are important for maintaining healthy bones, muscles, and overall physical well-being.

Physical fitness, in turn, also supports proper nourishment by helping to maintain a healthy body weight and composition. Regular exercise helps to increase muscle mass, which in turn increases metabolism, leading to improved energy balance and weight management. It also helps to reduce the risk of chronic diseases such as obesity, type 2 diabetes, and heart disease, which are all linked to poor nutrition and sea dentary lifestyle.

Furthermore, proper nourishment and regular physical activity also help to improve overall health and well-being, both physically and mentally. A well-nourished body with enough energy and nutrients can help to improve mood, reduce stress and anxiety, and increase overall feelings of well-being. Physical fitness also has positive effects on mental health, by releasing endorphins that can improve mood and reduce stress.

In summary, proper nourishment and physical fitness are closely linked, and they support each other. A well-nourished body with adequate physical activity results in optimal health and well-being, both physically and mentally. Nourishment can be considered a guide to physical fitness as it provides the body with the necessary nutrients to support and maintain optimal physical performance.

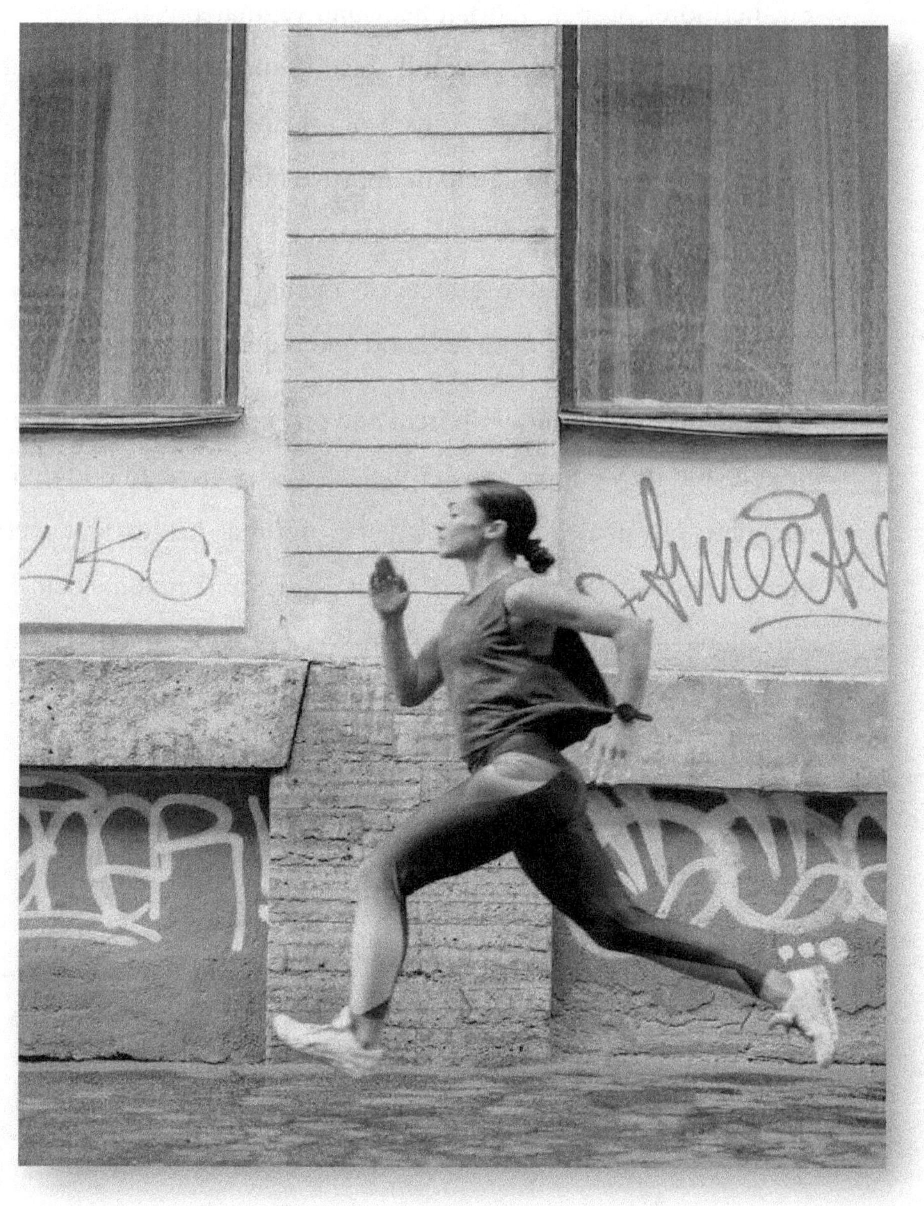

EXERCISE THAT PROMOTE HEALTHY LIFESTYLE

CHAPTER SIX

THE CONNECTION BETWEEN FOOD AND MENTAL HEALTH

Food is any substance that is consumed to provide the body with the energy and nutrients it needs to function properly. Food can be classified into several different categories based on its nutritional content and function, including carbohydrates, fats, proteins, vitamins, minerals, and water.

Carbohydrates, such as sugars and starches, are the body's primary source of energy. Fats, which are also a source of energy, provide the body with essential fatty acids and help to absorb certain vitamins. Proteins are important for the growth, repair, and maintenance of the body's tissues.

Vitamins and minerals are essential for maintaining healthy bones, muscles, and overall physical well-being. They are found in small amounts in food, and are sometimes referred to as "micronutrients."

Water is also considered a nutrient; it is essential for the body's metabolism and for maintaining proper hydration.

Food can be obtained from plants, animals, and other sources. Different cultures have their traditional foods, which can vary greatly in terms of ingredients, preparation methods, and nutritional content. It's important to have a balanced and diverse diet that includes a variety of nutrient-dense foods to support optimal health and well-being.

MENTAL HEALTH

Mental health refers to a person's general emotional happiness. It encompasses a wide range of emotional, psychological, and social well-being and it is an integral part of overall health and well-being.

A person with good mental health can cope with the normal stresses of life, work productively and fruitfully, and make a contribution to his or her community. They can maintain healthy relationships and have a sense of purpose and meaning in their lives.

FACTORS THAT CAN AFFECT MENTAL HEALTH INCLUDE:

Biological factors like heredities and mind interaction

Real Life experiences like suffering or abuse

Family history of mental health conditions

Personal habits and coping mechanisms

Socioeconomic status

Cultural and societal influences

Mental health conditions, such as depression, anxiety, bipolar disorder, schizophrenia, and eating disorders, are common and can affect anyone. They can be caused by a combination of genetic, environmental, and lifestyle factors.

Promoting mental health and preventing mental health conditions involves addressing the various factors that can affect mental health and providing support and care to those who need it. This can include things like therapy, medication, and support from friends, family, and the community.

It's also important to take care of oneself by getting enough sleep, eating a healthy diet, staying active and engaged in activities, practicing relaxation techniques, and maintaining a balance between work and leisure. Taking care of mental health is a continuous and ongoing process, and it's important to seek help if experiencing mental health challenges.

CONNECTION BETWEEN FOOD AND MENTAL HEALTH

There is a link between diet and mental health. The food we eat can have a significant impact on our physical and mental well-being.

A diet that is high in processed foods, added sugars, and saturated fats and low in fruits, vegetables, and whole grains have been linked to an improved risk of mental health conditions such as unhappiness and apprehension. A diet that lacks essential nutrients and vitamins can also contribute to mental health issues, as these nutrients are important for maintaining brain health and function.

On the other hand, a diet that is rich in fruits, vegetables, whole grains, lean proteins, and healthy fats, and that is also balanced, diverse, and moderate in energy intake, has been linked to improved mental health results.

 Studies have shown that a diet high in fruits and vegetables is linked to a lower risk of depression, while a diet high in omega-3 fatty acids, found in fish, nuts, and seeds, can improve symptoms of depression and anxiety.

A recent meta-analysis conducted by researchers at Linyi People's Hospital in Shandong, China, suggests that dietary patterns may play a significant role in the development of depression. The meta-analysis, which included studies from 10 different countries, found that there is a correlation between certain dietary patterns and the likelihood of developing depression. This supports the idea that what we eat can have a significant impact on our mental health.

Another study, led by Felice Jacka, Ph.D., the director of the Food and Mood Centre at Deakin University in Australia, found that dietary patterns are also related to the volume of the hippocampus in older adults. The hippocampus is a region of the brain that is important for memory and learning. The study found that individuals who followed a diet that was high in fruits, vegetables, and fish had a greater volume of the hippocampus compared to those who had a diet that was high in processed foods and sugar. This suggests that a healthy diet may help to protect the brain from the effects of aging.

It is important to note that these studies only suggest a correlation between dietary patterns and mental health and more research is needed to establish a causal relationship. However, the findings of these studies support the idea that a healthy diet can play an important role in maintaining good mental and cognitive health. It is always best to check with a healthcare expert before making any extreme changes to your food.

Proper hydration is also important for mental health, as dehydration can lead to fatigue and irritability, which can negatively affect mood. It is also important to note that eating disorders such as anorexia, bulimia, and binge eating can have a significant impact on mental health and can co-occur with other mental health conditions like despair and nervousness.

There is a sturdy that shows the connection between food and mental health. A diet that is high in nutrient-dense foods, such as fruits, vegetables, whole grains, and lean protein sources, has been linked to improved mood and cognitive function. Conversely, a diet that is high in processed foods, added sugars, and saturated fats have been associated with an increased risk of depression and other mental health conditions. Additionally, some specific nutrients, such as omega-3 fatty acids and vitamin D, have been shown to have a positive impact on mental health. Maintaining a balanced and healthy diet can have a positive impact on overall mental well-being.

Eating a balanced and healthy diet is crucial for maintaining good mental health. Studies have shown that a diet that is high in nutrient-dense foods, such as fruits, vegetables, whole grains, and lean protein sources, is associated with a lower risk of depression and other mental health conditions. These foods are rich in essential nutrients like vitamins, minerals, and antioxidants that are important for maintaining proper brain function.

Additionally, some specific nutrients have been found to have a positive impact on mental health. For example, omega-3 fatty acids, which are found in fatty fish like salmon and mackerel, have been shown to have anti-inflammatory effects and improve mood. Vitamin D, which is found in foods like eggs and fortified milk, is important for brain development and has been linked to a lower risk of depression.

On the other hand, a diet that is high in processed foods added sugars, and saturated fats have been associated with an increased risk of depression and other mental health conditions. These foods are often low in essential nutrients and high in calories, which can lead to weight gain and other health problems. Consuming too much sugar can also lead to blood sugar imbalances and contribute to mood swings, anxiety, and depression.

It's important to note that, diet alone cannot fully treat mental health issues, but it can be a complementary aspect to overall mental wellness. A combination of therapy, medication, and a healthy lifestyle can help improve mental health.

In summary, while the food we eat can't cure mental health conditions, it can play a role in maintaining and supporting mental well-being. Eating a balanced and nutritious diet that provides the body with the necessary energy and nutrients, and avoiding foods that may be detrimental to mental health is important for overall well-being. However, it's important to remember that mental health is multi-faceted and complex, and a healthy diet is just one aspect of it. It's important to consider other lifestyle factors, seek professional help when necessary, and consider a personalized approach to mental health care.

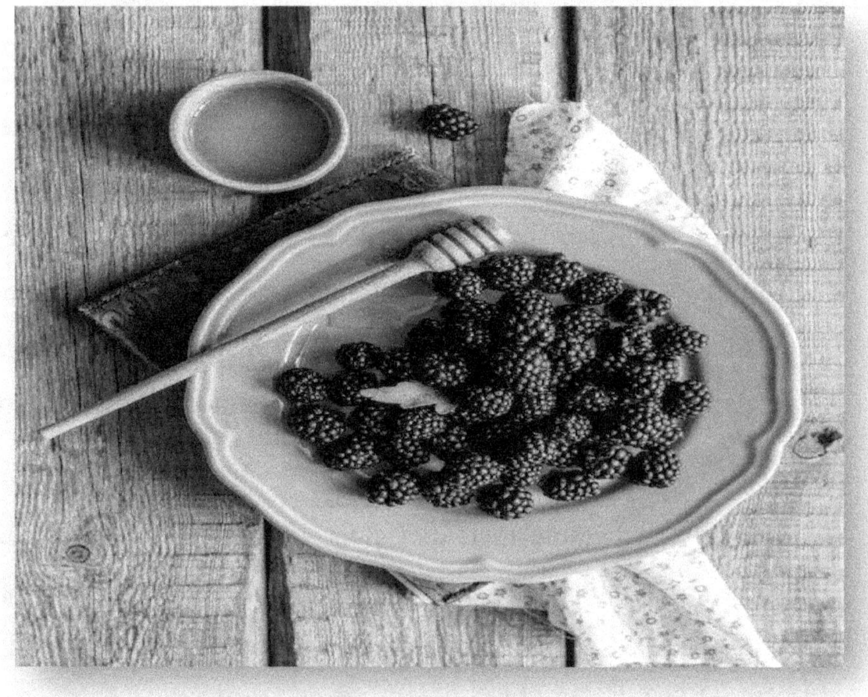

GOOD FOOD CAN ALSO HAVE EFFECT ON MENTAL HEALTH.

CHAPTER SEVEN

THE NOURISHMENT LIFESTYLE: HOW TO INCORPORATE HEALTHY HABITS INTO YOUR DAILY LIFE

A lifestyle is a way in which a person lives their life. It encompasses a wide range of factors, including personal habits, behaviors, and routines, as well as social and environmental factors that influence a person's overall well-being.

LIFESTYLE FACTORS THAT CAN AFFECT HEALTH AND WELL-BEING INCLUDE:

Diet and nutrition: The types and quantities of food and drink that a person consumes regularly can have a significant impact on their physical and mental health.

Physical activity and exercise: Regular physical activity and exercise can help to improve cardiovascular fitness, muscular fitness, and overall health.

Sleep: Getting enough quality sleep is essential for physical and mental well-being.

Stress management: Chronic stress can hurt physical and mental health, and it's important to have effective strategies to manage stress.

Smoking and alcohol consumption: These habits can have a significant impact on health and well-being.

Relationships and social support: Strong social support and positive relationships can have a positive impact on mental health.

Occupation and work-life balance: The nature of a person's work and the balance between work and leisure can also affect health and well-being.

Environmental factors: The physical and social environments in which a person lives can also affect their health and well-being.

HEALTHY AND NOURISHING LIFESTYLE

A healthy lifestyle involves adopting habits and behaviors that support overall well-being while avoiding those that can be harmful. It's important to note that everyone's lifestyle is unique, and what is considered healthy for one person may not be the same for another. It's also important to remember that lifestyle is a dynamic concept, it can change over time and it can be modified with effort and support.

A nourishing lifestyle supports optimal physical, mental, and emotional well-being by providing the body with the necessary energy and nutrients, and promoting healthy habits and behaviors. A nourishing lifestyle is focused on overall well-being, and it's not only about the food we eat but also the way we live.

A NOURISHING LIFESTYLE INCLUDES HABITS AND BEHAVIORS THAT SUPPORT OVERALL WELL-BEING SUCH AS:

Eating a balanced and diverse diet that is rich in whole, nutrient-dense foods and moderate in energy intake.

Staying active and engaging in regular physical activity.

Getting enough quality sleep.

Managing stress effectively through relaxation techniques and mindfulness practices.

Maintaining strong relationships and social support.

Finding a balance between work and leisure.

Engaging in activities that bring meaning and purpose to life.

Creating a safe and supportive environment.

Seeking professional help when necessary.

A nourishing lifestyle is not a one-size-fits-all approach, it's a personalized and dynamic concept that can change over time and adapt to different life stages and circumstances. It's a continuous and ongoing process of self-discovery, self-care, and self-improvement.

It's also important to note that a nourishing lifestyle is not a destination but a journey, and it requires ongoing effort and commitment. However, the benefits of a nourishing lifestyle are worth the effort, it can lead to improved physical and mental health, increased energy and vitality, and improved overall well-being.

Lifestyle can have a significant impact on healthy habits. A person's lifestyle can influence the types of behaviors and activities that they engage in regularly, which can in turn affect their overall health and well-being.

For example, a sedentary lifestyle that includes little physical activity and a lot of time spent sitting can make it more difficult to form healthy habits, such as regular exercise. On the other hand, an active lifestyle that includes regular physical activity can make it easier to maintain healthy habits, such as regular exercise.

Similarly, a diet high in processed foods and added sugars can make it more difficult to form healthy eating habits, while a diet that is rich in whole, nutrient-dense foods can make it easier to maintain healthy eating habits.

A lifestyle that includes high levels of stress can also make it more challenging to form and maintain healthy habits, such as stress management techniques. On the other hand, a lifestyle that includes effective stress management strategies can make it easier to maintain healthy habits related to stress management.

In summary, a person's lifestyle can have a significant impact on the formation and maintenance of healthy habits. A lifestyle that supports healthy behaviors and activities can make it easier to form and maintain healthy habits, while a lifestyle that makes it difficult to engage in healthy behaviors and activities can make it more challenging to form and maintain healthy habits. It's important to remember that habits are formed over time and with effort, and it's possible to make changes to one's lifestyle to support them.

Incorporating healthy habits into daily life can be challenging, but it is possible with a little bit of planning and effort.

TIPS TO HELP LIVE A HEALTHIER LIFESTYLE

Start small: It can be overwhelming to try to change too many things at once. Start by making small changes to your lifestyle and gradually build on them over time.

Make a plan: Set specific, measurable goals for yourself and create a plan to achieve them. Break your goals down into smaller, manageable steps and schedule them into your day.

Keep it simple: Try to find simple and sustainable solutions that are easy to incorporate into your daily routine. For example, choose a form of physical activity that you enjoy and that is easy to fit into your schedule.

Be consistent: Consistency is key when it comes to forming healthy habits. Try to make healthy behaviors a regular part of your daily routine, even if you can only do them for a short period.

Use reminders: Use reminders to help you stay on track, whether that's setting an alarm on your phone, putting a sticky note on your fridge, or using a planner to schedule your healthy habits.

Get support: Surround yourself with people who will support and encourage you in your efforts to form healthy habits.

Be flexible: Life can be unpredictable and it's important to be flexible and adaptable. Don't get discouraged if you slip up or miss a day. Just get back on your feet stronger and better.

Monitor your progress: Keep track of your progress and celebrate small wins along the way. This will help you stay inspired and make modifications where it is needed.

Remember, it's important to be patient with yourself and not to expect perfection. Incorporating healthy habits into daily life is a process and it takes time and effort, but the benefits are well worth it.

Here are some more practical steps you can take to incorporate healthy habits into your daily routine:

Wake up and go to bed at consistent times: Establishing a consistent sleep schedule can help regulate your body's internal clock and improve the quality of your sleep.

Plan your meals: Plan your meals and make sure they include a variety of nutrient-dense foods. Preparing healthy meals ahead of time can help you avoid last-minute decisions that lead to unhealthy choices. Incorporate physical activity into your day: Find an activity that you enjoy and that is easy to fit into your schedule, whether it's a morning walk, a lunchtime yoga class, or an evening swim.

Make use of reminders: Set reminders on your phone or computer to remind you to drink water, take a break from sitting or do a quick stretching routine.

Prioritize self-care: Make time for self-care activities such as meditation, journaling, or reading.

Make use of technology: Use apps, wearables, or other technology to track your progress and stay motivated.

Find a workout buddy: Exercising with a friend or family member can make it more enjoyable and help keep you accountable.

Keep healthy snacks on hand: Keep healthy snacks such as fruits, vegetables, nuts, and seeds readily available to help curb cravings and avoid unhealthy options.

Find ways to reduce stress: Find activities that help you relax and reduce stress such as yoga, breathing exercises, or listening to music.

Seek support: Don't hesitate to seek support from friends, family, or a professional if you need help incorporating healthy habits into your daily routine.

It's imperative to remember that everyone is unalike and what works for one individual may not work for another. Be patient with yourself and don't be afraid to experiment with different strategies until you find the ones that work best for you.

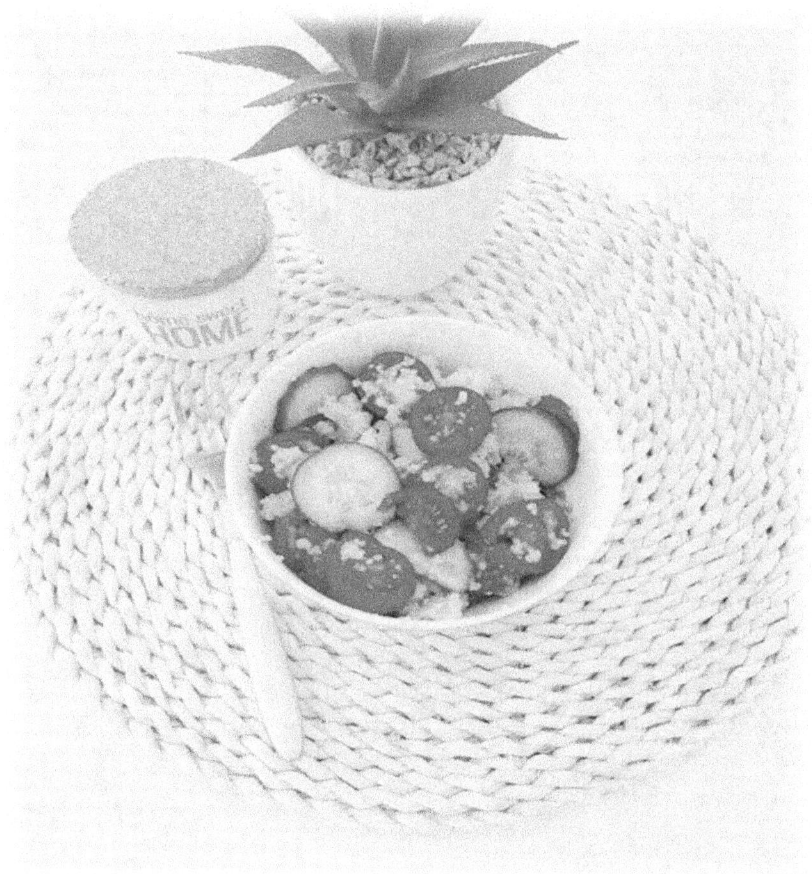